MW00884521

# FRUMPY
# TO
# FABULOUS

# ONE CHANGE A WEEK
# TO A HEALTHIER YOU!

# JOSETTE PUIG

Check off when you commit: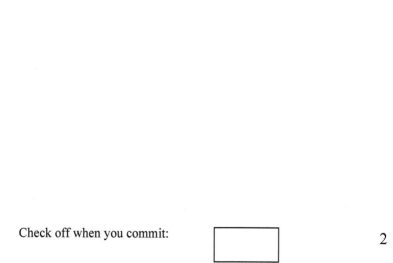

**Forward:**

I went on my first diet at age 10 and from then on I can honestly say I was always on some sort of diet. I tried them all and all I did was go up and down, then up and down again with no permanent results.

By the time I was 33 not only was I still overweight but I was depressed too. I was married and had 4 small children and I remember asking myself, "Is this it? Are my best years behind me?? Is my life just about keeping my head above water and taking anti-depressants??? What happened to me??!! I wanted more out of life. I wanted more for my children than just a mother who was existing. And then one day it all changed....

I read an article during the Christmas holidays of 2003 about how it takes 21 days to create new habits. I figured if I could just change my eating habits permanently I'd get real long-term results. But I also knew that making drastic changes would just overwhelm me, deprive me and drive me deeper into my depression.

On January 1, I sat down with a brand new 2004 calendar and decided I was going to make 1 change a week. That's it. Focus on that one change and add a new one each week. Four months later I was 30 pounds lighter, 6 months later I weaned off my medications and 52 weeks later I was a whole new person ready to live...REALLY LIVE!!!

Check off when you commit:

The following pages are a list of the changes I made week after week. You can use the boxes to check off each one as you make them. You may change the order but do not make more than 1 change a week. If you already do a few of these you may substitute for other changes/goals you want to achieve.
The point here is to not feel overwhelmed at any point and to embrace your new lifestyle habits.

You may feel that 52 changes is a long time but think about it, how have things turned out doing it your way?? And let's be honest, it takes time to create FABULOUSNESS!!
The best part about it is that year after year, it just keeps getting better! It's been 8 years since I made these changes and I can honestly say I continue to reverse the clock. Physically, mentally and emotionally. No diets, no pills, no shakes, no packaged foods, no fads, no gimmicks.
Its real food and real work. And now it's time to get real with yourself and Get Josette.

"The only thing standing between you and your goal is the bullshit story you keep telling yourself as to why you can't achieve it. ~ Jordan Belford

Check off when you commit:

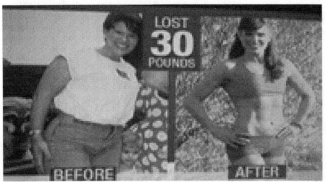

The weight has remained off.

Check off when you commit: ☐

## 2001

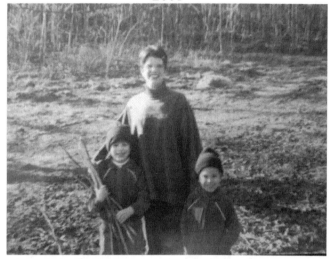

## 2011

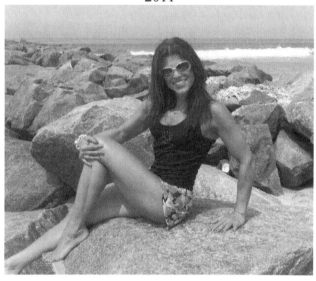

Check off when you commit:

Me and my 4 children

Check off when you commit: ☐

## SWITCH YOUR COFFEE CREAMER TO UNSWEETENED ALMOND MILK

Creamers and their fat-free versions are filled with artificial ingredients, sugar, calories and fat. Even low fat and skim milk are loaded with sugar. Many people don't realize this is the culprit to all-day sugar cravings. Don't kid yourself, those coffee drinks are really milkshakes with a shot of espresso! A 100 calorie reduction per day adds up to a 10 pound weight loss in 1 year.

This change alone is huge especially for those who drink more than 1 cup a day or take their creamer with a little coffee! Sugar is an inflammatory and suppresses our immune system too. It's no coincidence why flu season starts right after Halloween and goes on throughout Thanksgiving, Christmas and well into the New Year. Think about all the foods we consume during these holidays!

Check off when you commit:

## SWITCH WHITE BREAD TO WHEAT BREAD

\* All white starches get stored in your midsection creating the popular "muffin top"
White bread is refined to remove any healthy nutrients. It is chemically bleached and charged with gluten, salt and sugar.
White bread contributes to numerous digestive diseases, gluten allergies, type 2 Diabetes and obesity.
Read the labels on the packaging. Make sure the first ingredient says "whole wheat or whole grain."
If it says "enriched or unbleached" then it's been processed and it is not truly whole wheat.
*"The whiter the bread, the quicker you're dead!"* – old saying.

Check off when you commit:

WEEK 3

## BROWN RICE INSTEAD OF WHITE RICE

This may require an adjustment on your palate at first but each week your taste buds will become cleansed of your old diet habits (sugar and processed ingredients) and your new taste buds will embrace brown rice's hearty and nutty taste.

*White rice also contributes to "muffin top" syndrome
*White rice is processed from whole brown grain rice. The same type of thing as in brown bread vs. white bread scenario
*White rice converts to sugar which contributes to obesity and many health risk factors including Type 2 Diabetes
*Introduce it slowly to your family by making "half & half" batches of brown & white
*Each week use less white rice and in one month they'll be completely converted

Check off when you commit: 

10

# WEEK 4

## SWEET POTATOES AND YAMS INSTEAD OF WHITE POTATOES

White potatoes aren't necessarily unhealthy; it's their friends that make them naughty! (butter, sour cream, bacon bits, cheese)

*White potatoes have more sugar than Sweet Potatoes and Yams

*Consuming sugar will make you crave more sugar which gets stored as fat!! i.e...more muffin top!!

*Sweet potatoes and Yams are naturally sweet so you don't need to add all those extra calories and fats. i.e...butter, marshmallows, condensed milk

Check off when you commit:

WEEK 5

## **NONFAT GREEK YOGURT INSTEAD OF REGULAR**

Greek yogurt packs double the amount of protein than regular yogurt.
The straining process removes some of the milk sugar, lactose which may help those who are lactose intolerant.
Stay away from flavored yogurts which have added sugars, artificial sweeteners and carbohydrates.
Add fresh fruit, nuts and natural sweeteners such as Stevia to plain nonfat Greek yogurt for a healthy midmorning or bedtime snack.
Use Greek yogurt in recipes which call for mayonnaise or sour cream.

1 cup butter = 1/4 cup Greek yogurt + 1/2 cup butter
1 cup oil = 3/4 cup Greek yogurt
1 cup sour cream = 1 cup Greek yogurt
1 cup mayo = 1 cup Greek yogurt
1 cup cream cheese = 1 cup Greek yogurt
1 cup buttermilk = 2/3 cup Greek Yogurt + 1/3 cup buttermilk
1 cup heavy cream = 1/2 cup Greek yogurt + 1/2 cup heavy cream
1 cup milk = 1/4 cup Greek yogurt + 3/4 cup milk
1 cup fresh creme = 1 cup Greek yogurt

# WEEK 6

## PACK YOUR LUNCH AND SKIP THE DRIVE THRU

Let's be honest, do you REALLY know what's in that fast food burger or chicken? We've all heard the stories of how they make their "food" at these joints and if you haven't then it's time you know why fast food is cheap...BECAUSE IT'S CRAP!!! And if you eat crap you will LOOK like crap and FEEL like crap! And that's NOT FABULOUS!!!

*Control what you eat and how it's prepared
*Portion control – read your labels for the correct serving size
*Healthy food is not delivered through a drive thru window - Stop fooling yourself!
*Save money
*Eliminates guessing game. Deciding what to eat when you're starving is never a good idea

Check off when you commit:

## DRINK WATER

Water is to the human body like oil is to your car. Our bodies are made up of 70% water, and we lose two to three quarts of it every day through perspiration and other bodily functions. As a result, we need to constantly replenish our stores to ensure the right hydration levels to carry nutrients and waste to and from all our cells and organs, lubricate our joints, and regulate our body temperature.

A minimum of 64 ounces a day is good but you'll need more if you exercise and drink caffeine. A great way to make sure if you're having enough water is check the color of your urine. It should be see-through. So if it looks like apple juice, DRINK MORE WATER!

I tell my students, "If your pee is yellow, your energy will be mellow and your body will look like jello!!!"

You may feel the need to 'go' often when you increase your water intake but your body will adjust within a week.

Dehydration contributes to
*Lack of energy
*Constipation
*Hunger
*Headaches and migraines
*Cramps
*Bloating
*Weight gain
NONE of these are fabulous

Check off when you commit:

14

# WEEK 8

## GRILL IT OR BAKE IT

Fried foods not only make you fat but they are the leading causes of obesity and medical concerns. They age you inside and out!! Grilling and baking is not only a healthier option but a tastier one too! Let's be honest, EVERYTHING tastes better when it is hot off the grill! I use my George Foreman grill for those months when my outdoor grill is covered in snow.

*Less is more when you grill. You don't need heavy sauces or breading
*A little seasoning goes a long way with meats, chicken, vegetables, etc
*Grill a dozen chicken breasts and you'll have enough meals for the week such as salads, sandwiches or mixed with rice and beans

Check off when you commit:

## OLD FASHIONED OATS INSTEAD OF PACKAGED

Whether it's old fashioned or instant, the difference is how it's rolled and cooking time is shortened. Pre-packaged oats have added sugars and sodium.

My favorite way to cook oats is to add boiling water to oats and cover them, letting them set for 3-5 minutes. 1 part boiling water to 1 part rolled oats is a good ratio for starters. Add more or less water to suit your taste. I add cinnamon, berries and walnuts and a packet of Stevia to sweeten it.

*Quick cooking oats are the same except they've been cut down in size before being flattened to shorten cooking time
*Packaged oats have added sugars and sodium. Although convenient, they're not good for you
*Make your own travel packets. Portion oats into a plastic baggie and add your own flavorings. Keep them in your bag or at your desk. You can find a cup of hot water on a plane, airport, hotel...anywhere!
*I love the energy I get when I start my day with oatmeal. I feel AMAZING!!!!

Check off when you commit:

# WEEK 10

## SKIP THE CHEESE

When I tell my clients "cheese is mold", they say, "Ohhh but it's so good!" Then I say, "It's also one of the top contributors to cellulite! In fact, when I coach my fitness competitors it's one of the first changes I ask them to make in their diet and they're completely amazed at how fast they shed pounds and smooth their skin out.
I'm not saying swear off cheese for life but choose wisely! I will still have some on a whole wheat pizza but I 'feel' it the following day.

*Most cheese is processed and loaded with unhealthy fats. Not really a great source of protein
*The reduced fat versions are higher in sodium
*Non-fat versions have added artificial ingredients to make up for flavor
*About 75 percent of the world's population is genetically unable to properly digest dairy products, but most don't know this until they are off it
*Try giving up dairy for one week and watch your waistline, energy and digestive system improve

Check off when you commit:

## EXTRA VIRGIN OIL AND VINEGAR INSTEAD OF CREAMY DRESSINGS

This change alone can knock off 10 pounds in one year. Especially if you're more of a "I like salad with my dressing." A tablespoon of olive oil with balsamic or apple cider vinegar goes a long way.

*Bottled dressings have ingredients you can't even pronounce, which always mean it's no good for you
*Creamy dressings are loaded with fat, calories, sodium and sugar which only contribute to your waistline and arteries
*Olive oil is a healthy and 'healing' fat
*Olive oil helps fight heart disease, digestive illnesses, and many other illnesses
*Opt for Extra Virgin Olive oil which has been pressed once without using heat or chemicals. This oil is closest to its natural state

Check off when you commit:

## SAUTE WITH COCONUT OIL INSTEAD OF OLIVE OIL

Olive oil has many benefits but unfortunately loses its nutrients when cooking under high heat. Use it for drizzling your foods and dressings for your salad. Coconut oil used to be thought of as bad oil, high in saturated fat, but recent studies have shown that it actually helps you lose weight and has multiple health benefits too!
 Coconut oil maintains its nutrients under high heat and is great for sautéing meats and vegetables. A couple of teaspoons goes a long way too!

Health benefits of Coconut Oil include:
*Hair care
*Skin care
*Stress relief
*Maintaining cholesterol levels
*Weight loss
*Increased immunity
*Proper digestion and metabolism
*Heart disease
*Prevents high blood pressure
*Prevents cancer
*Thyroid and hormonal balance
*Kidney related illnesses
*Dental care
*Bone strength

Check off when you commit:

## SELTZER WATER INSTEAD OF SODA

Who doesn't love a bubbly drink? It's such a refreshing treat! But soda is a huge factor in obesity in this country, whether regular or diet, its poison to our bodies. Plus, drinking your calories is never a good idea. I'd rather eat my calories than drink them.

*Your goal should be to consume less than 25 grams of sugar per day
*A regular 12 oz can of soda has a whopping 39!!!!
*Diet soda has artificial sweeteners which are known to make you store body fat and increase your cravings
*Most sodas have caffeine which is a diuretic and cause dehydration making you even thirstier
*Seltzer water with a fresh lemon squeeze is a much healthier option and will help increase your water intake

Check off when you commit:

## NO MORE ARTIFICIAL SWEETENERS

Back in the 80's, Aspartame and Saccharin weren't such a
problem when we only had it in our coffee or an occasional diet
soda. But nowadays, everything has some form of sweetener
and we have proof that they contribute to many diseases as well
as obesity.

Artificial sweeteners create hormonal imbalances. Why is this
important? Because hormones are the messengers in our body,
They carry out signals to all parts of our body and tell it what to
do daily to keep it running healthy. Imagine a cop directing
traffic and suddenly becomes paralyzed in the middle of a busy
intersection. What do you think will happen? CHAOS!!!

My clients cannot believe the difference after they give up
artificial sweeteners, not just weight loss, but bloating, aches
and pains...it all goes away!!

Choose a natural sweetener like Stevia or even honey, agave,
sugar in the raw.

Now you understand why our bodies begin to shut down when
we turn 40; Our hormones get fed up from all the crazy diets,
packaged and artificial foods and they say "F-YOU! I'M NOT
GONNA LOSE AN OUNCE FOR YOU UNTIL YOU STOP
FEEDING ME CRAP"

Check your labels for Artificial Sweeteners such as:
yogurt, canned fruit, soda, bread, cereal, dressings, cookies,
dips, juice, popcorn, snack bars, gum, jello, pudding, ice cream
shakes, vitamins

Check off when you commit:

## ALCOHOL AND ITS SLIPPERY SLOPE

Research shows 4-6 ounces of red wine a day has many benefits but let's be honest, who actually measures their wine every time?

This is one most of my clients don't want to hear but excessive alcohol will keep you from shedding weight and feeling fabulous.

*Increases blood sugars

*Makes you retain body fat and water

*Increases appetite. One of the reasons there are daily happy hours at assisted living homes is because most elderly tend to lose their appetites as they get older. (Something to look forward to I guess)

*Decreases inhibitions which may lead to poor food choices. We've all been there. A few too many drinks at a party only to wake up the next day and not remember what you ate the entire night

*"The Hangover" meal is never a healthy one

*Although alcohol may be effective in sleep induction, it impairs sleep during the second half of the night and can lead to a reduction in overall sleep time. Have you ever seen an alcoholic look well-rested?

Check off when you commit:

## CHOOSE YOUR MORNING CEREAL WISELY

Many cereals make claims of extra fiber, protein, vitamins and nutrients. Don't fall for them until you read the labels. These are usually hiding extra sugars, sodium and artificial ingredients.
Here are a few suggestions I recommend.

*Cheerios
*Shredded Wheat
*Fiber One
*Grape Nuts

Check off when you commit:

## EAT BREAKFAST WITHIN 30 MINUTES OF WAKING UP

A well-balanced breakfast of lean proteins, healthy fats and complex carbohydrates boosts metabolism, provides energy and helps you avoid binging all day.

"But I'm not hungry!" is not a good excuse; that tells me you have a slow metabolism, which only leads to storing more fat when you do get around to eating, that's how Sumo wrestlers are trained. They don't eat until lunch hour so they're able store calories and gain weight, which is why most Americans are looking more and more like Sumo wrestlers these days.
Eat breakfast within 30 minutes of rising to fuel your mind, body and spirit.

*Whole grain cereal and skim milk or unsweetened almond milk
*Scrambled egg whites and whole wheat toast
*Oatmeal & a scoop of protein powder with berries
*Wheat toast & all natural almond butter drizzled with honey
*Whole wheat French toast
*Greek yogurt with fresh berries & walnuts
*Protein Pancake (GetJosettte.com/en/recipes)

Check off when you commit:

24

# WEEK 18

## EAT EVERY 2-3 HOURS

This is an important factor for me, not just for my waistline, but to keep my energy up and my mind clear all day long. I was able to get off antidepressant pills by choosing the right foods and fueling my brain continuously. If I waited too long to have a meal or a snack it would mess with my emotional balance.

Eat small and frequent meals 5 or 6 times a day to maintain blood sugar levels preventing you from hunger.
*Keep metabolism working. (Again, to avoid the Sumo Wrestler physique)
*Never allow yourself to get to starvation. This leads to overeating and poor food choices
*Keep energy levels high all day long
*Build muscle and burn fat with a revved up metabolism
* Control your mood by fueling you body, mind and spirit throughout the day

Check off when you commit:

## KEEP NON - PERISHABLE HEALTHY SNACKS IN YOUR CAR

This will keep you from doing those mindless drive thru window runs or eating your kids' snacks.
Remember, it's not food if it's delivered through a window.
Keep these portioned and tucked away in the trunk of your car to keep you from mindless eating.

*Wheat crackers
*Almonds
*Rice cakes
*Tuna pouches
*Protein powder
*Oatmeal
*Peanut butter or almond butter

## CHOOSE RAW ALMONDS AND WALNUTS OVER PEANUTS

Stay away from all those roasted and glazed nuts which are loaded with sugar and salt. Choose nuts with healthy fats which will help you lose weight too!

*Higher in Omega 3s and 6s.
*Portion control. Measure them into snack bags before diving into the bag as it is very easy to get carried away.
- Just because they're good for you doesn't mean "all-you-can-eat"
*Fight off hunger, leaving you fuller
*Almonds
*Walnuts
*Pistachios
*Make your own trail mix by mixing these with dried fruit but make sure those don't have any added sugar either

Check off when you commit:

## CONSUME STARCHY CARBOHYDRATES WITH PROTEIN AT BREAKFAST, LUNCH AND DINNER

*Choose from wheat bread, brown rice, oatmeal, sweet potato, yams, red bliss potatoes, whole wheat pasta, and quinoa. Staggering these at breakfast, lunch and dinner will keep your energy and mood elevated throughout the day.
And of course, you can always add fruits and vegetables to these meals.

*Turkey sandwich with an apple
*Oatmeal with berries and scrambled egg whites
*Grilled chicken with brown rice and black beans and spinach salad
*Lean beef with sweet potato and asparagus
*Whole wheat pasta with turkey meatballs
*Natural peanut butter, jelly and banana on whole wheat wrap

Check off when you commit:

## CONSUME SIMPLE CARBOHYDRATES WITH PROTEIN FOR SNACKS

Fruits and vegetables will keep your energy up in between meals and keep your blood sugars from dropping which can lead to binging.

*Apple with natural peanut butter
*Green pepper slices with hummus
*Greek yogurt with berries & walnuts
*Carrot sticks and nuts
*Turkey & avocado lettuce wraps
*Tuna salad made with Greek yogurt, walnuts & apples

Check off when you commit:

## 1 TREAT MEAL A WEEK

A sweet a week is a treat. A sweet a day is a habit.

A treat meal a week will keep you on track when you know you have something to look forward to at the end of the week. What can you have?? Eat what you've been craving without any guilt but keep it to that one meal and then go back to your routine. I love to indulge in wine, a big bar burger with sweet potato fries and ice cream for dessert. Yes...all in one sitting!! Increasing your caloric intake one day a week is also good for weight loss. This forces your thyroid to release a hormone which signals your body to work harder. Of course, this only works when you do it once a week.

*Choose one day of the week and circle it on your calendar
*Plan your treat meal around a social engagement if you want
*No deprivation here
*Make sure you exercise on your treat meal day to rev up your metabolism

Check off when you commit:

## AVOID THE "MAKE IT PIZZA NIGHT" PITFALL

We all have those hectic nights, running around with kids, activities and late-night meetings, but unless you're making your own whole wheat pizza crust and adding healthy ingredients to it, ordering pizza may be an occasional easy fix but not for your waistline.

*Keep 3-5 phone numbers of restaurants you know that prepare healthy meals on your speed dial
*Keep restaurant menus in your car, so you may commit to your order before dialing
*Keep easy meal ideas in your freezer. A pound of frozen shrimp and veggies is faster to whip up into a stir fry than waiting for pizza
*Every dinner doesn't have to be an event, sometimes a protein shake and a salad is exactly what your body needs
 *Breakfast for dinner is always an easy solution too
Scrambled egg whites with spinach and peppers with a couple slice of whole wheat bread

Check off when you commit:

WEEK 25

## READ FOOD LABELS

In order to be fabulous you must also become educated in the art of reading nutrition labels. Supermarkets don't want you to know all the hidden garbage that keeps you addicted to shopping at their stores but you have a right to know. Become an expert nutrition label reader and don't ever trust the front of a box. In addition, Smartphones have an application called 'Fooducate', which you can scan food items with and it will help you make healthier food choices. Take it with you next time you shop….AMAZING!!!

*A healthy food label normally has 5 ingredients or less
*If a 3rd grader can't pronounce it, you shouldn't eat it
*The first ingredient is what it contains most of in the package
*1 gram of fat = 9 calories
*1 gram of carbohydrates = 4 calories
*1 gram of protein = 4 calories
*Check sugar content. We shouldn't consume more than 25 grams/day from packaged foods
*Watch out for Low-fat and Fat free products, they have added sugar, sodium and artificial ingredients

Check off when you commit:

## WEEK 26

## HELP! I JUST ATE AND I'M STILL HUNGRY!

Let's face it; we eat when we're bored, happy, stressed, and sad. Figure out what other things you can do to keep your mind occupied. I taught myself how to knit because my brain doesn't receive the "I'm full signal" as often, so I figured knitting would keep both hands occupied. It reduces my urge to snack and it relaxes me too.

Here are some other ideas
*Take a walk
*Go for a bike ride
*Hit the gym
*Shopping
*Get a pedicure
*Stretch
*Give yourself a manicure
*Fold laundry
*Shower
*Brush your teeth
*Pick up a book
*Help your children with their homework
*Give your dog a bath

Check off when you commit:

WEEK 27

## MOVE! MOVE! MOVE!

The human body was meant to move...EVERYDAY!! I don't care what you do but you must move! Keep a boom box in the kitchen and dance while you're fixing dinner! YES! It's that easy!! Exercise does NOT have to be grueling like you see on TV. Just get started and do it consistently!
You can't look fabulous if you don't feel fabulous and exercise releases endorphins which is our body's own 'happy pill'!!

*Dance
*Swim
*Walk
*Run
*Lift
*Stretch
*Buddy up with a co-worker or friend to keep each other motivated
*Take the stairs
*Take your phone calls standing up while you're at work
*Do something at the top of every hour

My website has great videos to give you ideas and keep you motivated at home or at your office.
www.GetJosette.com

Check off when you commit:

34

# RESEARCH YOUR RESTAURANTS BEFORE DINING OUT

Study the restaurant menu online and decide what you'll order before you leave your home. Don't wing it! Chances are you'll be hungry by the time you sit to order and that's never a wise time to choose.

*If you know a restaurant serves large portions, request they pack up half of it before they place your food on the table
*Be prepared to ask your server to request any changes to your order. You'd be amazed how accommodating servers are when you ask nicely
*Avoid All-You-Can-Eat Buffets. Just cause it says so doesn't mean you should
*Split entrees and desserts. Sometimes all you need is a few bites to feel satisfied

Check off when you commit:

## WEED RECOGNITION

Weed Recognition (cut off people who don't support your lifestyle)
Some people want to see you succeed and others want to see you fail. We all have those friends who say they support us but as soon as we start to look and feel good they say "So, how much longer are you going to do this diet thing?" You tell them "I'm not on a diet, I eat healthy."

I've seen this one here cost many marriages and friendships but you must realize life is about growing. On my road to getting fabulous I've learned your friends can be anchors or engines...the choice is yours!

*If they don't support you then you need to cut them out
*If it's important to you, it should be important to them
*Taking control of your health so you're not a burden to others in the future
*Choosing a healthy lifestyle to set an example to your children
*I feel as an organ donor it is my duty to take care of my body so someday I can help others attain better health
*Your body is your permanent home. Raise the rent and evict those not willing to pay

Check off when you commit:

WEEK 30

# DO NOT REWARD YOURSELF WITH FOOD YOU'RE NOT A DOG

There are many ways to reward yourself along your fitness journey. Here are a few ideas.

*Take progress photos every 4 weeks
*Treat yourself to a new pair of sneakers
*New workout clothes will keep you motivated to hit the gym
*Host a healthy dinner party. Have your friends bring fit versions of the usual foods and exchange recipe cards
*Try a new workout like Hot Yoga or Boot Camp or dance class
*Treat yourself to a weekend spa vacation

Check off when you commit:

37

# WEEK 31

## SWITCH ENERGY DRINKS FOR WATER

People consume energy drinks for a quick morning boost, or an afternoon pick-me-up. The problem is the crash that comes with it, makes you crave another jolt, which is exactly what the makers of these products want...YOU addicted to THEIR product!

All of these trendy drinks are filled with sugar, artificial ingredients and caffeine. Caffeine and some of these ingredients are diuretics, which mean they dehydrate your body. In essence, they're sucking out all of your 'natural' energy since the human body is 70% water.

Next time you feel tired, drink 16 ounces of water, it'll do a much healthier job perking you up.

Check off when you commit:

## CREATE YOUR OWN HAPPY HOUR

Who says happy hour must include alcohol and appetizers?
Why not create your own "Healthy Happy Hour" tradition??

*Grab a group of girls and try a new fitness class at a local
studio
*Host a workout DVD swap party! Your old workout might be
exactly what your friend is looking for!
*Host a workout clothes swap! Just leave behind the worn out
stuff
*Exchange your favorite healthy recipes
*Long walks with your BFF are better than therapy

Check off when you commit:      

## SKIP THE VENDING MACHINE

There's nothing healthy that comes out of a vending machine. Even prepackaged trail mix has added sugar and salt. Bring your own snacks to work, your children's soccer games or anytime you step out of the house.

*Wheat crackers & natural peanut butter
*Greek yogurt & fruit
*Green pepper slices & hummus
*Apples & tuna
*Homemade trail mix (almonds, walnuts, craisins)
*Get Josette Bar - you can find the recipe on www.getjosette.com

Check off when you commit:

WEEK 34

## SKIP FROZEN MEALS FOR PREPARED LEFTOVERS

The invention of the T.V. dinner unraveled digestive illnesses, obesity, Type 2 Diabetes and many other diseases. Not surprising considering these meals are filled with artificial flavors, colors and fillers to extend their shelf life. Unfortunately these shorten your shelf life!
The so-called 'Healthy" versions of these are just as bad.

*Prepare extra portions and store leftovers in plastic containers
*Ground turkey
*Chicken
*Brown rice
*Sweet potatoes
*Vegetables

Check off when you commit:

41

# WEEK 35

## COOK IN BULK - PORTION AND STORE IN PLASTIC CONTAINERS

Carve out 2 hours a week to do this. It may seem like a lot of time in the kitchen but it ends up being far less than cooking a meal each night. And not having to think about what you're making for dinner each night too. I love to prepare 2-3 meals in separate crock-pots, then portion and store them in the freezer.

*Chicken
*Brown rice
*Black beans
*Sweet potatoes
*Cut fruits an veggies for snacks
*Prepare snacks like crackers & peanut butter
*Trail mix

Check off when you commit:

WEEK 36

## TRY A NEW RECIPE EACH WEEK

Keep it simple!

Some of the best and healthiest recipes are actually very easy.
There are plenty of places you can pick up new recipes or ideas
on improving your traditional ones into healthier versions. My
video website will show you delicious, nutritious and easy
recipes you and your family will love!

*www.GetJosette.com
*Friends
*Magazines
*Healthy food websites
*Supermarket

Check off when you commit:

43

## SHOP WITH A LIST

You've heard "Don't go grocery shopping hungry." Well, I'm adding "Don't go shopping without a list!" Shopping hungry and without a list always equals disaster. You over-shop, over-spend and buy crap your body doesn't need.

*Make a weekly meal plan
*Make a daily meal plan
*Stay on the peripherals of the supermarket
*Avoid the inner aisles of the store
*Organic doesn't always mean it's healthier. An organic "toaster pastry" is still filled with artificial ingredients
*If you eat the peel buy organic
*Choose grass fed and hormone free animal protein

Print our Clean Eating grocery list at:
http://getjosette.com/en/downloads

Check off when you commit:

## LAY OUT OR PACK UP YOUR WORKOUT CLOTHES BEFORE YOU GO TO BED

By doing this, you eliminate any excuse to skip your workout the next day.
If you wait to do this, you will make every excuse to procrastinate putting yourself first: from work, laundry, phone calls, appointments, emergencies, you name it.

Packing your bag or putting on your workout clothes before leaving your bedroom will automatically increase your energy and focus.

This only takes 5 minutes but it's one of the biggest things that will dictate your mood. Let's face it, you never regret going to the gym but you'll always regret skipping it.

Check off when you commit:

## MAKE A WORKOUT PLAYLIST

Music has the power to energize you, motivate you, and inspire you. It can also bring you down to tears. Create a song list you know will get in your head, under your skin and feel it in your blood.

Don't limit yourself! This is a great way to expand your music library!
*New songs
*Old school music
*Borrow a friend's playlist to get ideas
*Try different rhythms. Latin music has great and upbeat sounds
*Choose songs with inspiring lyrics
*Exchange IPods with your kids to keep you up on the most current tunes

Check off when you commit:

## PORTION CONTROL

Even though you may be eating really healthy by now, over-scooping your portions may keep you from losing those last 5-10 pounds. This is the time you must get real with your portions and measure your food.
A short person doesn't eat as much as a tall one. Females require fewer calories than males. Athletes and fitness enthusiasts require more fuel than those who do not exercise. Know your portions. Here are some great tools that will help keep you in check.

*Electronic food scale - This is the best tool I've ever used
Better than any gym membership
*Measuring cups
*Measuring spoons
*Use smaller bowls & plates (dinner plates used to be 9-inches, now they average 13!)

Check off when you commit:

# WEEK 41

## CONSUME PRE AND POST WORKOUT MEALS

Your body is at its weakest right after your workout so you must give it proper nutrients so it may replenish and rebuild. Your pre and post workout meals are just as important as your workout and if you want results from your exercise regiment, you must fuel your body properly.

Pre workout - Eating Whole grains, protein and good fats will give you great energy for your entire workout. This can be consumed 1-2 hours prior to exercise
*Oatmeal & egg whites
*Protein pancake with berries
*Whole wheat toast with natural peanut butter and banana slices
*Turkey sandwich on whole wheat
*Greek yogurt with berries and nuts
*Granola bar
*Get Josette Bar

Ideas for post workout - Limit fats in your post workout meal because they will slow the absorption of protein to your muscles. You need a fast digesting protein and carbohydrate here.
This should be consumed within 30 minutes of your workout
*8 ounces of skim chocolate milk
*Protein shake with berries
*Greek yogurt with fruit

Check off when you commit:

## KEEP A FOOD JOURNAL

I will not see a client unless they keep a food journal. I tell them "If you bite it, you write it." It's that simple. In order for me to help them, I need them to get real with themselves. Keep yourself accountable by tracking the foods you eat. It keeps you in check when you're falling off the weight-loss wagon. This will make you think twice before stopping at your coworker's desk for an extra piece of candy.

My website has an online tool which provides easy food logging, recipes and community support. I have a great tool on my website called FatSecret and you can find it at www.GetJosette.com

Other options are
*Carry a small notebook
*Smartphone applications like My Fitness Pal or Calorie Tracker

Check off when you commit:

WEEK 43

## SWITCH POTATO CHIPS TO WHOLE GRAIN CRACKERS

Potato chips and even their so-called 'healthy' baked chips are filled with trans fats, sodium and artificial ingredients. If you want a salty crunch, grab a wheat cracker.
If you think this transition is too difficult then you're always welcome to make it slow.

*Switch from regular chips to baked chips
*Once your bag of baked chips runs out replace it with healthy whole wheat crackers
*Make your own sweet potato skins or kale chips! I have these easy recipe videos on my website, www.Getjosette.com

Check off when you commit:

## WEIGHT TRAIN 3 TIMES A WEEK

Research shows the importance of weight training especially as we get older. Our bodies produce their own calcium when we lift and it helps fight Osteoporosis.
Ladies, you won't look like Arnold if you lift heavy weights. I laugh when I hear ladies say, "I don't want to get big" as they lug around 30 pound babies in their car seat carrier, then they throw equally heavy strollers in the trunk of their SUVs and then they don't want to lift a 20 pound dumbbell??

If you've never ventured into a weight room, hire a trainer for a few sessions or tag along with a fit friend to help you get acclimated. There are also group fitness training classes but I must stress to you to go at your own pace and DO NOT lift to the beat of music!

*Aim for 3 times a week. It can be a full body circuit or you can break it down in body parts
*Strength training increases metabolism and burns fat longer than cardiovascular exercise
*Only way to change your body composition
*Muscle is more dense than fat
*I used to be a size 12 but now I'm a 2 with only a 20 pound weight loss
*Increases bone density
*Strong is the new Sexy

Check off when you commit:

## SKIP THE "ALL YOU CAN EAT FOR $7.95" BUFFET

Just because it says it, doesn't mean you should! Think about what's in these foods!
Most are sitting in oils, breading, sauces and tons of salt until they're prepared.
Then, to make matters worse, as if 1 plate of this crap isn't bad enough, you go back for more!!
3,500 calories can go down very quickly at these joints. In fact, you could leave 5 pounds heavier between all the fat and sodium loaded foods. This type of eating could take weeks to clean up. So not worth it!!


*There's a reason it's ALL-YOU-CAN-EAT for $7.95. The quality of the ingredients aren't worthy of your hard-earned healthy body
*3,500 calories = 1 pound = 20 minutes at a buffet
*With big plates and the ability to endlessly refill them, portion control becomes a losing battle
*You never feel fabulous once you've eaten here

Check off when you commit:

## Set your alarm 20 minutes earlier

Rising just 20 minutes earlier will help:
*Get your cooler packed for the day
*Dinner plans figured out
*Workout clothes in your gym bag and loaded to your car
*Put your game face on. A little makeup goes a long way to feeling fabulous
*Rushing through your morning routine can frazzle your entire day and lead to emotional eating to calm your nerves

Check off when you commit:

## MAKE A SMART BEVERAGE SWAP

Coffee drinks, flavored waters, juices, sodas, energy drinks....Having these everyday can add up to plenty of empty calories. Whether you have 5 or 50 pounds to lose, it's never a good idea to drink your calories.

I understand these are special treats for some of you but remember, once a week is a treat, once a day is a habit and these little habits add up quickly especially if you're trying to lose those last pesky 10 pounds.

*Decide on having one every other day
*Next week commit to having only 1 during the week and circle it on your calendar
*You'll notice your energy increase, waistline decrease and save a lot of money!
*In 2010 I brewed my coffee for an entire year. I saved $1,460!! I took myself on a cruise for my 40th birthday with that money

Check off when you commit:

54

## SWITCH YOUR BEDTIME SNACK

People have the misconception that you shouldn't eat before going to bed. Truth is calories don't know what time it is and it's important to nourish your body.

*Greek yogurt with crushed walnuts
*Low fat cottage cheese with berries
*Apple slices with natural peanut butter
*Air-popped popcorn

Check off when you commit:

## EAT HORMONE FREE ANIMAL PROTEIN

Many food producers use corn feed, growth hormones and antibiotics to feed their livestock to help speed up their time to market, which means we end up consuming these growth hormones and antibiotics. YUCK!!
Grass-fed beef is richer in heart-healthy omega-3 fats, while its corn-fed counterparts are loaded up with excess omega-6 fats, which counteract the benefits of omega-3s.

Protein is involved in every part of your body, from your bone marrow to your skin.
*We need high-quality protein at almost every meal
*Protein that has not been contaminated by chemicals, pesticides, growth hormones or antibiotics
*Proteins are found in both animal and vegetable sources
*Animal-source protein is complete protein because almost all animal proteins contain all eight essential amino acids in optimal proportions

Check off when you commit:

## DON'T GIVE UP

"The Drop Effect" is a term used to describe when your body doesn't show any weight loss on the scale for approximately 4 weeks. This can be a very frustrating time for those of us who are being so diligent with our food and exercise programs. In fact, most of us quit right before this!
For those of you who haven't quit at this point...BRAVO and you will be happy to know that your body is simply going through major body composition changes during this time. Soon after the four week mark you'll be surprised to see the changes in how your clothes fit, the numbers on the scale, and most importantly, how you feel. This is a huge incentive to stay on track and keep plugging away.
Unfortunately most of us never experience the drop effect because we believe in all these quick weight-loss gimmicks. The drop effect is the big payout for those who are truly serious about taking control of their health.

Check off when you commit:

# WEEK 51

## PMS WEEK CAN BE YOUR FAT LOSS WEEK

The week before you get your menstrual cycle, PMS week, you retain 5 pounds of water, feel tired, lethargic, sore breasts, feel fat and you just want to wear oversized sweat pants and give into your cravings. This is actually the optimal time when the female body burns most fat. YES!!! Your body releases its own fat burner hormone during this week.

This is the time you need to be more focused than ever and push through your workouts even harder. DO NOT sabotage this time with mindless eating. If you stay focused and disciplined you will make huge strides towards your fitness goals and you will see and feel the difference after your cycle is over.

How your period affects your workout: Averaged on a 28-day cycle

Day 1-12: You should aim for speedier cardio. Fast and intense workouts seem easier thanks to high estrogen levels.

Day 13-15: Estrogen plummets and muscles get less oxygen causing your mind and motivation to slow down.

Day 16-28: Long steady cardio sessions are recommended. Estrogen begins to creep back but progesterone which triggers the body to store fat and retain water in case of pregnancy is dominant. Go longer and steady pace to beat the bloat!

## KEEP IT FUN!!

If eating healthy and being fit weren't fun, I wouldn't do it!
Trust me. Starving and grueling exercise is never fun but eating
in moderation and dancing for exercise is!!
Do whatever it takes to keep the "fun" in fitness! Sign up for
walks, 5ks, marathons, dance classes. Step out of your comfort
zone and try something completely scary!! For some that may
be a hip hop class...maybe try kickboxing or martial arts.
Challenge your body with diet and exercise.
Once you change your approach to food all of these changes
will become lifetime habits.

*Empower yourself
*Strengthen your mind, body and spirit
*More energy
*Better and balanced mood
*Hormonal balance
*Increase libido
*Set a great example to your family


Remember, food is medicine. It can give you life, or suck the
life out of you.


Check off when you commit:

## ACKNOWLEDGMENTS

I'd like to thank my friends and family who have been so incredibly supportive of my journey and always believed in me. I also want to thank my fiancé, my soul mate and business partner Chris Macrina. You give me wings when I need to fly and ground me when I need to focus. But above all, for loving me just the way I am. I love you....Always and Forever!!

Check off when you commit:

# Website

Be sure to join our website www.GetJosette.com

Check off when you commit:

## Disclaimer:

PLEASE NOTE: Always consult a physician before starting a fitness program or changing your diet. Information found in this book is meant to support and not replace the relationship with your physician. Not all exercises or activities are suitable for everyone. If you feel discomfort or pain, stop. The instructions and advice presented are in no way intended as a substitute for medical or psychological counseling.

By reading this book or accessing Get Josette, LLC (NOTE that Get Josette, LLC refers to the web site itself, www.getjosette.com, Get Josette, LLC , and anyone associated with the site, either through giving advice, writing articles and providing content), you certify that you have received consent from your physician to participate in the programs, workouts, and exercises to be provided by Get Josette, LLC

© 2012, Josette Puig & Get Josette, LLC
Self publishing
(To contact Josette Puig or Get Josette, LLC please email admin@getjosette.com)

**ALL RIGHTS RESERVED**. This book contains material protected under International and Federal Copyright Laws and Treaties. Any unauthorized reprint or use of this material is prohibited. No part of this book may be reproduced or transmitted in any form or by any means, electronic or mechanical, including photocopying, recording, or by any information storage and retrieval system without express written permission from the author / publisher.

Check off when you commit:

14768006R00033

Made in the USA
Charleston, SC
29 September 2012